CARLAT PUBLISHING

Treating Alcohol Use Disorder

A Fact Book

Daniel J. Carlat, MD

Publisher, Carlat Publishing
Associate Clinical Professor, Tufts University School of Medicine
Boston, MA

Michael Weaver, MD, DFASAM

Professor of Psychiatry, University of Texas
Health Science Center, Houston, TX
Medical Director, Center for Neurobehavioral Research on Addiction

Talia Puzantian, PharmD, BCPP

Professor, Keck Graduate Institute School of Pharmacy
Claremont, CA

Published by Carlat Publishing, LLC
PO Box 626, Newburyport, MA 01950

CARLAT PUBLISHING

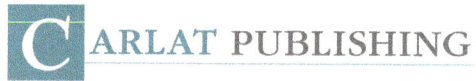

Published by Carlat Publishing, LLC
PO Box 626, Newburyport, MA 01950

Publisher and Editor-in-Chief: Daniel J. Carlat, MD
Deputy Editor: Talia Puzantian, PharmD, BCPP
Senior Editor: Ilana Fogelson
Associate Editor: Harmony Zambrano

This CME/CE activity is intended for psychiatrists, developmental and behavioral pediatricians, psychiatric nurses, psychologists, and other health care professionals, including primary care providers, with an interest in mental health. The Carlat CME Institute is accredited by the Accreditation Council for Continuing Medical Education to provide continuing medical education for physicians. The Carlat CME Institute maintains responsibility for this program and its content. The Carlat CME Institute designates this enduring material educational activity for a maximum of six (6) *AMA PRA Category 1 Credits*™. Physicians should claim credit commensurate only with the extent of their participation in the activity. CME quizzes must be taken online at www.thecarlatreport.com.

To order, visit www.thecarlatreport.com
or call (866) 348-9279

ISBN #:
Print - 979-8-9873354-2-0
eBook - 979-8-9873354-3-7

PRINTED IN THE UNITED STATES OF AMERICA

NOTES FROM THE AUTHORS

The goal of these fact sheets is to provide need-to-know information (on a single page) that can be easily and quickly absorbed and utilized during a busy day of seeing patients.

Cost information. We obtained pricing information for a one-month supply of a common dosing regimen from the website GoodRx (www.goodrx.com), accessed in January 2023. These are the prices patients would have to pay if they had no insurance (GoodRx also offers coupons to purchase certain medications at reduced prices). Because of wide variations in price depending on the pharmacy, we list price categories rather than the price in dollars. The categories are: $: Inexpensive (<$50/month); $$: Moderately expensive ($50–$100/month); $$$: Expensive ($100–$200/month); $$$$: Very expensive ($200–$500/month); $$$$$: Extremely expensive ($500/month).

ACKNOWLEDGEMENT
We thank the following experts who have reviewed portions of the manuscript: Bachaar Arnaout, MD; Joao P. De Aquino, MD; Robert Blake Werner, MD; Noah Capurso, MD.

FINANCIAL DISCLOSURES
Dr. Carlat, Dr. Weaver, and Dr. Puzantian have disclosed that they have no relevant relationships or financial interests in any commercial company pertaining to the information provided in this book.

DISCLAIMER
The information in this book was formulated with a reasonable standard of care and in conformity with current professional standards in the field of psychiatry. Treatment decisions are complex, and you should use these fact sheets as only one of many possible sources of medical information. Please refer to the PDR (Physicians' Desk Reference) when you need more in-depth information on medications. This information is not a substitute for informed medical care. This book is intended for use by licensed professionals only.

If you have any comments or corrections, please let us know by writing to us at info@thecarlatreport.com or The Carlat Psychiatry Report, P.O. Box 626, Newburyport, MA 01950.

Table of Contents

Alcohol: An Overview

The Basics

Composition: Alcohol, also known as ethanol, is the byproduct of the metabolism of any starch or sugar with the addition of yeast. The resultant chemical, CH_3CH_2OH, is an ethyl group linked to a hydroxyl group (hence the term "ethanol").

Prevalence: Alcohol is the most widely misused substance. Currently, 90% of US men and 70% of US women consume some form of alcohol, though most of them do not consume large amounts. In any given month, 23% of Americans binge drink, and 6% drink heavily.

Mechanism: Alcohol acts rapidly because it is very lipid soluble. Cell membranes, with their lipid bilayers, offer almost no impediment to it. Alcohol's effects on the gamma-aminobutyric acid (GABA) receptor lead to its psychoactive effects, though we don't precisely know the biochemical mechanism of intoxication.

Intoxication: At low to moderate doses, alcohol creates relaxation and disinhibition. However, with greater consumption, alcohol affects deeper brain structures, causing sedation and amnesia ("blackouts") and ultimately affecting the respiratory drive.

Assessment for Alcohol Use Disorder (AUD)

Assessment includes a standard diagnostic interview that focuses on uncovering alcohol use issues (see "Alcohol Use Disorder: Initial Evaluation Template" and "Alcohol Use Disorder: Tips for the Initial Assessment"), determining how many DSM-5 AUD criteria are met (see "How to Ask DSM-5 Focused Questions for Alcohol Use Disorder"), reviewing labs, and assessing for any medical issues (see "Medical Issues and Alcohol Use Disorder").

Psychosocial Consequences

Alcohol use and intoxication can additionally lead to the following:

- Impact of DUI (driving under the influence charge), including deaths and injuries
- Poor decision making while under the influence
- Loss of interest in hobbies or anything other than alcohol (ie, anhedonia, avolition)
- Secondary psychiatric complications

Withdrawal

Withdrawal symptoms typically begin six to eight hours after the last drink and last 24–48 hours. They can include:

- Autonomic hyperactivity (sweating or pulse >100 bpm, elevated temperature, elevated blood pressure)
- Increased hand tremor (also tongue fasciculations)
- Insomnia
- Nausea or vomiting
- Transient visual, tactile, or auditory hallucinations
- Psychomotor agitation
- Anxiety
- Generalized tonic-clonic seizures

Treatment

Treatment is divided into short term (medically guided withdrawal management) and long term (psychotherapy and long-term medication treatment). Withdrawal symptoms can be life-threatening (see "Alcohol Withdrawal Time Course and Symptoms") and there are several detox protocols to choose from, depending on the detox setting (see "How to Manage Alcohol Withdrawal in Outpatient Settings" and "How to Manage Alcohol Withdrawal in Inpatient Settings"). Long-term treatment entails motivational interviewing (see "Motivational Interviewing in Alcohol Use Disorder"), encouraging participation in 12-step programs (see "Alcoholics Anonymous Meetings: The Basics"), and use of medications such as naltrexone, acamprosate, or disulfiram (see fact sheets for each; we've also assembled versions you can hand out to patients).

In this book's medication fact sheets, the notation **[G]** indicates that a medication is available in generic as well as branded options.

Interesting Fact

Most yeasts cannot grow in alcohol concentrations greater than 18% by volume. This creates a natural limit to the strength of fermented beverages like wine and beer.

Alcohol Use Disorder Assessment

Alcohol Use Disorder: Initial Evaluation Template

Introduction

This template can be downloaded and adapted for your charting, or you can use it as a guide to remind you of important topics to cover during the initial interview.

Identifying Data

History of Present Illness (Focused on Alcohol Use)

- Age at first use
- Pattern of current use (type of alcohol, quantity, and frequency)
- Period of heaviest use
- Negative consequences
- Longest period of sobriety
- History of treatment
    - 12-step programs
    - Individual and/or group therapy
    - Medications (naltrexone, acamprosate, disulfiram, etc.)
    - Inpatient/residential
    - Sober housing (halfway house)

Other Substance Use History

Past Psychiatric History (Non-Substance Use Disorders)

Social History

Medical History

- General
- Alcohol-related
    - Liver disease, heart disease, hypertension, peripheral neuropathy
    - Exams: Skin for jaundice and spider angioma, neuro for tremor and dementia

Labs

- Complete blood count for anemia, macrocytosis
- Comprehensive metabolic panel for electrolytes, kidney function
- Liver function tests
- Vitamin deficiencies, including folate, thiamine, pyridoxine
- Urine tox screen
- Blood alcohol level

Mental Status Exam

Assessment

Plan

Alcohol Use Disorder: Tips for the Initial Assessment

Introduction

This fact sheet suggests a typical flow of questions during a conversational initial assessment of a patient's alcohol use. While many of these questions can be used to establish a DSM-5 alcohol use disorder diagnosis, they are not explicitly tied to the DSM-5 criteria. To conduct a more formal interview based on the DSM-5, see "How to Ask DSM-5 Focused Questions in Alcohol Use Disorder."

Initial Questions

Start with a nonthreatening question like, "Do you have a drink now and then?"

If the patient's response is, "I don't drink," it's possible they are part of the 15%–20% of people who do not drink. If so, follow up by determining the reason for not drinking (often it's due to a bad family experience with alcohol). Sometimes this response doesn't mean that the patient never drinks, but simply indicates that they don't drink often.

"How often do you typically drink?" You can also include a gentle assumption in this question, such as, "How often do you drink—daily? A few times a week?"

Assessing Consumption and Withdrawal Risk

"How much have you been drinking in the last two to four weeks? Has your drinking gone up or down recently?" Patients who have been drinking consistently and heavily for four weeks or more are at higher risk of alcohol withdrawal symptoms.

"What has been your longest period of abstinence? Have you been able to go for several days without a drink in the last six or 12 months?"

"Have you been through alcohol withdrawal before?" This question helps you to assess the chances that the patient will go into withdrawal in the future. If the patient doesn't know what withdrawal means, use specific phrasing such as, "If you go without a drink for a day or two, do you get shaky or sweaty?"

Assessing Consequences of Drinking

"Have bad things happened to you as a result of drinking? Have you experienced any legal consequences, like a DUI? Have you had any relationship problems because of drinking? Have you lost any jobs?"

In our experience, patients don't always realize the negative consequences of their drinking. For example, a patient's alcohol use may have led to a divorce, but unless the ex-spouse made the reason for the split clear, the patient might not be aware of it. Other examples of consequences that may not be so obvious include:

- Not speaking to one's children for a prolonged period, perhaps because when the parent is drunk, the kids don't enjoy the interaction
- Not being allowed to see grandchildren (or nieces or nephews) because the parents of the children don't want to risk that the patient will be drinking then
- Changing jobs frequently, possibly as a result of poor performance caused by frequent hangovers
- Having a friend group consisting solely of drinking buddies

Assessing History of Treatment

"Have you done anything to try to quit drinking? Have you gone to AA meetings? Have you taken any meds like naltrexone, disulfiram (Antabuse), or acamprosate? Have you had counseling sessions?"

"Have you ever been in the hospital for drinking problems, like in a detox unit? Have you been to rehab? Have you lived in a sober (halfway) house?"

"What was the most effective thing you've done to quit drinking?"

Single Screening Question

Validated screening questions are less useful in psychiatric practices since we have more time to spend discussing things with patients, but they are useful for busy primary care practices.

"How many times in the past year have you had X or more drinks on one occasion?" (where X = 5 for men and 4 for women). Once in the past year is considered positive and requires further assessment of drinking.

How to Ask DSM-5 Focused Questions for Alcohol Use Disorder

Introduction

Alcohol use disorder (AUD), as defined in the DSM-5, includes 11 criteria. While most experienced clinicians can diagnose AUD without going through a formal checklist of DSM symptoms, we suggest you try using this sheet during interviews. You are likely to find it helpful in at least two ways.

First, you can use the criteria to more accurately categorize the severity of your patient's AUD:

- Mild: two DSM-5 criteria
- Moderate: three to five DSM-5 criteria
- Severe: more than five DSM-5 criteria

Second, you can use the criteria to show your patient that there are relatively objective medical symptoms leading to the diagnosis of AUD. This lessens the stigma attached to the diagnosis and shows that you are a well-trained professional, enhancing your credibility and hopefully helping your patient trust your recommendations.

Below, we suggest questions for each of the 11 criteria. Although the DSM-5 doesn't explicitly divide the criteria into categories, we find it helpful to do so, and below we list them under four broad clusters: impairment of control, social consequences, risky behavior, and tolerance/withdrawal.

Questions About Time Spent Obtaining Alcohol (Impairment of Control)

1. *Cravings:* "Do you have cravings (urges to drink)?"
2. *Using more than planned:* "Do you often drink more than you really want to or intend to?"
3. *Unable to quit despite attempts to do so:* "Have you tried to cut down or quit drinking before?" "What is the longest time you have been abstinent? How long ago was that?"
4. *Significant time spent obtaining or recovering from alcohol:* "How often do you go to the liquor store?" "How long do you spend at the bar?" "How many hours per day do you avoid family or work because of drinking or recovering from drinking?"

Questions About Activities Given Up Over Time Due to Drinking (Social Consequences)

5. *Activities given up due to drinking:* "Are you spending less time with your family than before?" "Have you avoided going out because you prefer to stay home to drink?"
6. *Failure to fulfill major role obligations:* "Have you had to take time off from work because of drinking?" "Have you called in sick to work after drinking?"
7. *Persistent social and interpersonal problems:* "How much time do you spend socializing in settings that don't involve alcohol? Is this less time than before?" "Do you have arguments with friends or family due to drinking?" "Have you lost friends?"

Questions About Use in Hazardous Situations (Risky Behavior)

8. *Recurrent use in physically hazardous situations:* "Have you ever driven after drinking? Have you ever had a DUI charge? Have you ever had a charge for being drunk in a public place (public intoxication)? Have you ever drank while on the job?"
9. *Continued use despite knowledge of negative consequences:* "Have you continued to drink after a doctor told you about medical problems caused by drinking?"

Questions About Tolerance and Withdrawal

10. *Tolerance:* "Do you need to drink more than you previously did to get a buzz or to get drunk?"
11. *Withdrawal:* "Have you been through alcohol withdrawal before?" "Have you had problems getting to sleep after drinking?"

Blood Alcohol Level Fact Sheet

Introduction

Blood alcohol level (BAL, sometimes called BAC for blood alcohol concentration) is often used in emergency rooms to give insight into the severity of a patient's alcohol use and to help guide predictions about when they will be sober enough for a psychiatric evaluation and when they may start to experience withdrawal.

How Is BAL Measured?

BAL is the percentage of alcohol in a person's blood, usually expressed as grams per deciliter (a deciliter is one-tenth of a liter, or 100 milliliters). For example, a BAL of 0.1% means there is 0.1 gram of alcohol per 100 milliliters of blood. Most clinical settings prefer to express BAL as milligrams per deciliter (mg/dL), in which case the previous percentage is multiplied by 1000. This makes communicating BAL easier since you don't have to use fractions—for example, instead of saying, "His BAL is 0.1%," you can say, "His BAL is 100." In this fact sheet, we will express BAL as mg/dL.

BAL Facts

- The US and Canada define legal intoxication—at which point it is illegal to drive—as a BAL of 80.
- Most people will become visibly intoxicated above a BAL of 100. However, those with a lot of tolerance may still appear sober at 150 or above.
- One standard drink increases BAL by 20–40, depending on factors such as sex and weight. Legal intoxication generally requires three to four drinks consumed within about an hour.
- The body can metabolize 10–15 mg/dL of alcohol per hour, but chronic drinkers metabolize it faster, around 20–30 mg/dL per hour. A rule of thumb is that the liver can metabolize about one standard drink per hour.
- A patient's BAL does not help in determining when they will go into withdrawal. While one might assume that withdrawal correlates with a very low BAL, in fact many patients with severe alcohol use disorder drink so regularly that they "live" at a BAL of 400–500 and will often begin to have withdrawal symptoms at a BAL of 200 or higher.

Factors Affecting BAL

- *Weight:* Given the same consumption of alcohol, heavier individuals will have a lower BAL than lighter individuals.
- *Sex:* Men metabolize alcohol at a faster rate than women, so men will have a lower BAL given the same consumption.
- *Speed of drinking:* The faster people drink, the higher their BAL.
- *Alcohol and food:* Drinking on an empty stomach increases absorption, leading to a quicker increase in BAL.

How BAL Is Used Clinically

- To determine when a patient is "sober enough" to be evaluated by psychiatric clinicians. It's common for psychiatric services to require that a patient's BAL be lower than 200 before they conduct an interview. Sometimes, insurance companies will also require a low BAL before they will cover a psychiatric evaluation.
- To evaluate the causes of extreme agitation or sedation in patients who are unable to communicate their history. In these cases, blood is drawn for many tests, including a BAL, in order to document that alcohol is or is not related to the presentation.

How to Order Biomarkers of Alcohol Use Disorder

Introduction

Biomarkers of alcohol use are sometimes helpful when we are not sure whether our patients are reliable in reporting their level of use. Here are two common situations where we might order a test:

- Screening for ongoing alcohol use in a patient who is requesting controlled substance medications for a psychiatric issue
- Monitoring for relapse in a patient who has been abstinent and who is in a mandated treatment program (such as part of probation or an employer-mandated program)

Screening for Recent Use/Relapse

These tests screen for alcohol directly. They are useful for detecting whether a patient has consumed alcohol within the last few hours.

- *Blood alcohol level (BAL):* BAL is mainly used in emergency room settings (see "Blood Alcohol Level Fact Sheet" for details). Time window for detection: First appears 15 minutes after use, detectable for six to 10 hours.
- *Urine alcohol content (UAC):* UAC can be measured in the emergency room, is less invasive to measure, and can be assessed serially. It peaks 45–60 minutes after ingestion and is about 1.3 times the BAL. Time window for detection: Appears one hour after use, detectable for nine to 12 hours.
- *Breathalyzer:* Breath testing results are directly normed to the BAL and similarly give an indication of degree of intoxication. Newer developments include smartphone apps with attached breathalyzers that allow patients or family members to do BAL testing (various devices are available on Amazon.com for around $100). Time window for detection: Appears one hour after use, detectable for 12–24 hours.
- *Ethyl glucuronide (ETG) and ethyl sulfide (ETS):* ETG and ETS are metabolites of alcohol that remain in the urine for two to three days after drinking. These tests are more sensitive and have a longer time window than either urine alcohol content or a breathalyzer test. They are considered the gold standard for assessing whether a patient has had a drink over the past few days.

Screening for Chronic Use

The following common blood tests are indirect markers of alcohol use. They are useful in determining that a patient likely has been a heavy drinker, but they aren't as reliable and specific as other tests regarding the time course of drinking.

- *Gamma-glutamyl transferase (GGT):* GGT is a glycoenzyme on endothelial cell membranes of various organs, especially the liver. Increased levels of GGT generally indicate that a patient has been drinking heavily and continuously for several weeks. Since GGT levels take two to six weeks to normalize, patients will need a decent length of sobriety before producing a normal GGT.
- *Carbohydrate-deficient transferrin (CDT):* CDT is a more specific blood test than GGT and is good for detecting chronic heavy drinking as opposed to moderate drinking. Transferrin is an iron transport protein that loses some of its carbohydrate side-chains in the presence of alcohol. Thus, the specific "carbohydrate-deficient" transferrin indicates alcohol use. Only prolonged heavy drinking (ie, greater than four or five drinks a day for two to three weeks), however, is likely to produce an elevated CDT level. So, although this test is well suited to identify heavy drinkers, it is not good for detecting relapse or moderate drinking. This test is more specific to alcohol use than the GGT test.
- *Aspartate amino transferase (AST) and alanine amino transferase (ALT):* Elevations in AST and ALT may reflect liver damage caused by alcohol. An AST:ALT ratio of 2:1 is more indicative of alcohol-induced liver damage compared to other sources of liver injury. However, this measure is not as specific to drinking as GGT.
- *Mean corpuscular volume (MCV):* Chronic heavy alcohol use can cause MCV elevation both because of alcohol's detrimental effect on erythroblast development and as a secondary effect of vitamin deficiencies sometimes seen in severe alcohol use disorder. This test is not as sensitive to alcohol use as other biomarkers.

Medical Issues and Alcohol Use Disorder

Introduction

While you will not be treating most medical complications of alcohol use, it's important to ask patients about these things, especially as part of the motivational interviewing strategy. Identifying significant medical sequelae during an interview can be a powerful incentive for patients to consider the negative consequences of drinking. In essence, this comprehensive medical survey will help to "scare them sober."

Common Alcohol-Related Complications and Questions to Ask

- *Cardiovascular:* Hypertension, cardiomyopathy, arrhythmias: "Have you had any chest pain or palpitations?"
- *Gastritis and bleeding:* "Have you had ulcers? Have you ever noticed dark stools or blood in your stool?"
- *Liver injury (hepatitis and cirrhosis):* "Have you had belly pain, especially on your right side, after drinking heavily? Have you had yellow eyes (jaundice)?"
- *Low levels of clotting factors due to liver disease:* "Do you have a tendency to bruise or bleed easily?"
- *Neuropathy:* "Have you noticed numbness or tingling in your feet?"
- *Dementia:* "Have you had memory or concentration problems?"
- *Anemia:* "Has your energy level or stamina been low?"

Labs to Order (see table for more comprehensive list)

- *Liver function tests:* Alanine and aspartate transaminases (ALT and AST). Elevation of these enzymes is caused by leakage from damaged liver cells. Mild elevations (less than four times the upper limit of normal) are common and usually reversible with abstinence. Elevations of four or more times the upper limit of normal (usually >200 depending on the lab) are most concerning (they indicate acute alcohol-induced hepatitis).
- *Coagulation studies:* Prothrombin time (PT) or international normalized ratio (INR). Elevation in these results indicates more serious liver damage. In such a state, the liver is so damaged that it is not making coagulation factors, and a person will bruise easily due to "thin" blood that doesn't clot well.
- *Complete blood count (CBC):* Anemia may be caused by the direct toxic effect of alcohol on bone marrow, or by low levels of thiamine, folate, and vitamin B12 due to drinking. This is usually reversible with abstinence and adequate nutrition; patients don't generally need to be on vitamin supplementation long term.

Labs for Medical Consequences of Alcohol Use

Lab Type	Effect in Alcohol Use Disorder
Markers of Liver Inflammation	
Alanine transaminase (ALT)	More elevated in non-alcoholic fatty liver
Aspartate transaminase (AST)	More elevated in alcoholic liver disease
Gamma-glutamyl transferase (GGT)	Most sensitive for alcoholic liver disease
Markers of Liver Synthetic Function Problems	
Albumin	Decreased in alcoholic liver disease
Direct bilirubin	Increased in alcoholic liver disease
Indirect bilirubin	Increased in alcoholic liver disease and malnutrition
Prothrombin time or international normalized ratio (INR)	Increased in alcoholic liver disease
Other Relevant Labs	
Iron panel	Iron accumulates in alcoholic liver disease
Hematocrit	Decreased in anemia
Mean corpuscular volume	Elevation indicative of B12 deficiency
Platelet count	Decreased in alcoholic liver disease
White blood cell count	Decreased in alcoholic liver disease

Alcohol Use Disorder Treatment

Alcohol Use Disorder Treatment: An Overview

Introduction

There are many approaches to treating alcohol use disorder (AUD), and the initial approach for any given patient will vary depending on the severity of their use, their experience with treatment, the existence of concurrent illness, etc. This fact sheet gives you a framework for choosing an initial treatment strategy based on how many of the 11 DSM-5 criteria for AUD the patient meets.

Mild AUD (Two DSM-5 Criteria)

Typical scenario: The patient sometimes drinks more than planned, occasionally missing work or social obligations due to drinking.

- Simple advice/brief therapy to aid in self-tapering (eg: "Try cutting down on your own. Start by going from three beers per day to two or two and a half, and so on until you've stopped.")
- Self-help resources: National Institute on Alcohol Abuse and Alcoholism website (www.niaaa.nih.gov); self-help books, such as *Alcohol Lied to Me* by Craig Beck and *The 10-Day Alcohol Detox Plan* by Lewis David (refer patients to Amazon.com to browse many other options)

Moderate AUD (Three to Five DSM-5 Criteria)

Typical scenario: The patient often drinks heavily, has tried to quit in the past, and has had significant psychosocial consequences, but is still able to maintain a relatively functional family or work life.

- Psychotherapy with a certified substance use disorder therapist
- Alcoholics Anonymous (AA) meetings
- Possible medication treatment

Severe AUD (More Than Five DSM-5 Criteria)

Typical scenario: The patient's life revolves around drinking; they have had significant health/legal consequences and have found it difficult to hold a job or maintain relationships.

- Frequent AA meetings
- Intensive outpatient program
- Medication treatment
- Inpatient rehabilitation facility
- Sober house

Alcohol Use Disorder: Psychosocial Treatment Options

Introduction

There are many effective nonpharmacological treatments for alcohol use disorder (AUD). In this fact sheet, we provide an overview of the major options. You may be able to conduct some of these treatments yourself (such as motivational interviewing), while in other cases you will refer the patient to others. This is a helpful list to have by your side, especially when your patient is not responding to your usual treatments.

Psychotherapy

- *Cognitive behavioral therapy (CBT):* Teaches patients to recognize and avoid situations that provoke alcohol cravings; it also teaches strategies to cope with cravings, such as distraction, recall of negative consequences, and positive thought substitution. CBT can be quite effective in patients who stick to treatment and who consistently practice coping skills.
- *Motivational interviewing (MI):* A brief patient-centered approach that aims to help patients identify and resolve ambivalence about changing their drinking patterns in a collaborative and nonjudgmental manner.
- *12-step facilitation (TSF):* Like Alcoholics Anonymous (AA), TSF promotes abstinence and is based on the idea that alcohol misuse is a spiritual and medical disease. TSF involves weekly sessions assessing a patient's alcohol use, attendance and participation in AA meetings, and setting goals for engagement in AA.
- *Alcohol behavioral couples therapy (ABCT):* Outpatient treatment that includes a patient's partner in weekly sessions spanning 12–20 weeks. ABCT takes a CBT approach to identifying behaviors that trigger and reinforce alcohol use. It supports change though increasing positive couple interactions, adopting coping skills to promote abstinence, and using positive reinforcement to modify behaviors.

Behavioral Treatment

- *Contingency management (CM):* CM is also known as voucher-based reinforcement therapy (VBRT). It rewards patients for behaviors consistent with sobriety, such as providing consecutive negative urine tox screens or having good attendance at treatment sessions. The rewards are usually gift certificates or lottery tickets but are sometimes cash. The more consecutive negative samples submitted, the greater the reward. In one study, adding VBRT to standard behavioral therapy doubled participants' duration of abstinence (from six weeks to 12 weeks).

Mutual Self-Help

- *Alcoholics Anonymous (AA):* Free meetings, run by volunteers, that are based on the AA 12-step approach. AA is generally considered the most effective treatment for AUD, at least for patients who are motivated to participate fully.
- *Self-Management and Recovery Training (SMART Recovery):* Mutual-help meetings that are an alternative to AA and based more on principles of CBT and MI than on 12 steps. They are also free, and meetings are in person or virtual. (www.smartrecovery.org)
- *Secular Organizations for Sobriety:* Another alternative to AA that uses nine principles instead of 12 steps and deliberately does not have a spiritual or religious focus compared to AA. (www.sossobriety.org)

Clinic-Based Treatment

- *Intensive outpatient program (IOP):* Generally provided in a format of nine hours per week spread over three days. Components include individual sessions, group sessions, psychoeducational sessions, and strong encouragement to attend 12-step programs. Two large studies have compared different intensities of IOP with "standard" treatment such as four or six hours per week of therapy sessions, and both programs were equally effective. This implies that as long as patients are participating in some significant therapeutic treatment, they are likely to improve.

Online Treatment

- *Moderate Drinking (MD):* A subscription-based patient-oriented approach toward monitoring alcohol intake based on principles of behavioral self-control training. There are a variety of smartphone applications (apps) that promote recovery and provide tracking of number of sober days, AA meeting locators, journaling options, and links to other resources. Some are free, while others require an activation fee. Examples include Sober Buddy, I Am Sober, Dry Days, and Sober Grid.

How to Quickly Develop a Therapeutic Alliance

Introduction

Regardless of what kind of treatment you choose for your patient, it's important to remind yourself of the key feature of any successful treatment—a good treatment alliance. Here are some of the tried-and-true basics.

- Sit down to speak with the patient, rather than standing up while you talk (relevant primarily with inpatient treatment settings where you are visiting patient rooms). This communicates that you are carving out time to understand the patient.
- Make eye contact with the patient while you talk, rather than spending the majority of your time looking through the medical record.
- Use empathetic statements during every visit.
  - "That sounds difficult."
  - "I can understand why you're struggling."
  - "You've done a great job simply surviving your childhood."
- Rather than starting the interview by asking about alcohol use, start by showing interest in the patient as a person.
  - "Before we get into why you were admitted here (or why you made this appointment), tell me a little about yourself."
  - "How is your life? What do you do for a living? Where do you live?"
  - "Who's important in your life? What are some of your goals? What kinds of things do you like to do for fun?"
- Be nonthreatening and nonjudgmental in your approach.
  - "Would you be comfortable telling me a little bit about your history of issues with alcohol? I understand you've had some struggles with that at times."
- Try to understand positive aspects of the patient's use. Don't come across as the naïve clinician who ignores that people use alcohol because it makes them feel good. Don't automatically assume there is a negative explanation for the patient's use, such as irresponsibly wanting to get wasted. Acknowledge that people often use because it improves mood, relieves boredom, enhances their ability to socialize with others, or allows them to stick with a challenging or menial job.
  - "What is it that you like most about using alcohol? How does it help you deal with stuff in your life?"
- Confront the issue of stigma head-on. Is there a history of trauma? Is the underlying psychiatric disorder the key driver? Is there a chronic pain issue? Convey respect and explicitly battle stigma.
  - "I've worked in the addiction field long enough to know that stigma is a big deal for a lot of my patients."
  - "I'm a human and you're a human, and I want to understand your pain so I can help you."

Motivational Interviewing in Alcohol Use Disorder

Introduction

The goal of motivational interviewing is to enhance your patient's motivation to decrease their alcohol intake. The technique focuses on working with the patient wherever they are in the process of change. Rather than telling them to change, you are always listening for signs of their own internal motivation.

RULE Mnemonic—The Therapist's Mindset

- *R:* Resist telling your patient what to do—instead, use the interview to help them create their own solutions.
- *U:* Understand your patient's motivation.
- *L:* Listen to your patient with empathy.
- *E:* Empower your patient to set achievable goals and to overcome barriers.

"Good Things and Less-Good Things" Method

1. Start by asking, "Tell me some of the good things about drinking." They will enumerate the various positive aspects, such as, "It relaxes me; it gives me something to do when I'm bored."
2. Then ask, "OK, are there any less-good things about drinking?" They might say, "When I drink I don't do things that I should be doing, like cleaning up the house or looking for a job."
3. Summarize what you've heard: "So it sounds like drinking can be positive because it helps you feel less anxious and it gives you something to do when you're bored. But on the other hand, it makes you forget to do some things you want to do, like cleaning the house or looking for a job. Did I get that right?"
4. Explore the patient's motivation to change: "Do you think there are more positives to drinking, or more negatives?" This will lead to a discussion that helps them understand whether they want to moderate or stop drinking.

"A Typical Day" Method

This is a particularly good technique for patients who are not very talkative. It's also a good general question for beginning your alcohol use evaluation.

1. Say, "Walk me through a typical day of yours, starting from when you get up."
2. As your patient answers, listen for whether they volunteer information about how drinking may be causing problems for them. For example, they might say, "I usually have a glass of wine around 4. I try not to start drinking any earlier because then I can't get any more work done." Then you can reflect back: "So drinking sometimes interferes with your work? Tell me more about that."
3. Even if the patient doesn't mention alcohol at all, this can still provide an opportunity. You can say, "I noticed that you didn't mention alcohol at all during a typical day. Please help me understand where alcohol fits in." Then reflect back on issues that arise.

Assess Readiness to Change

Once you've identified that your patient has some motivation to quit, ask about their readiness to change. One technique is to use the "readiness ruler."

- Start by asking, "On this scale from 1 to 10, where 1 is definitely not ready to change and 10 is definitely ready, what number best reflects how ready you are to cut down?" Then ask why they didn't choose a lower number. This results in the patient providing reasons for why they are more likely to change, called "change talk" or self-motivational statements.
- Then ask, "On the same scale, how confident are you that you can cut down?"

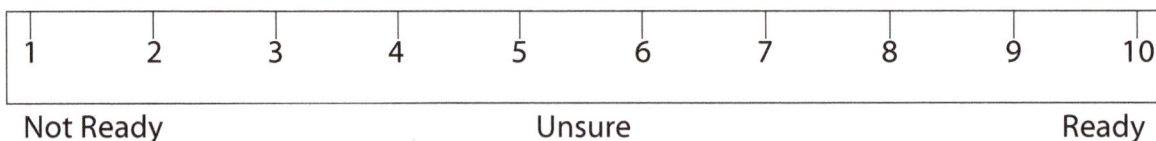

1	2	3	4	5	6	7	8	9	10
Not Ready				Unsure				Ready	

Start the Treatment Process

Once you've established that your patient is motivated to cut down, you can start discussing treatment options/recommendations, such as Alcoholics Anonymous meetings (see "Alcoholics Anonymous Meetings: The Basics"), identifying triggers (see "Teaching Relapse Prevention Techniques in Alcohol Use Disorder"), medication-assisted treatment (see "How to Choose the Right Medications for Alcohol Use Disorder"), and so on.

Cognitive Behavioral Therapy Techniques in Alcohol Use Disorder

Introduction

Cognitive behavioral therapy (CBT) is highly effective for alcohol use disorder (AUD) patients—but only if they are motivated and determined to complete homework exercises and to practice assigned coping skills. Many clinicians naturally use CBT techniques with AUD patients without knowing it. For example, any time you discuss relapse prevention strategies (see "Teaching Relapse Prevention Techniques in Alcohol Use Disorder"), you are using a version of CBT.

Overall Strategy

It's difficult to control our behaviors without knowing how our thoughts and emotions lead to those behaviors. CBT helps patients unravel the chain of automatic negative thoughts that lead to negative emotions, which in turn lead to drinking behaviors. You will teach your patient strategies for questioning and changing thoughts, improving emotional responses, and finding ways to avoid negative behaviors.

Identify a Specific Drinking Episode to Begin Analysis

Start by briefly educating your patient about the CBT technique and get their consent to do this work. Then, ask them to recount a recent drinking episode: "Let's try to figure out what we can learn from what happened. Tell me more about the situation and what led you to drink."

For each situation, identify:

- Automatic negative thoughts (ANTs)
- Emotions
- Actions
- Rational positive responses

See "Automatic Negative Thought Worksheet for Cognitive Behavioral Therapy" for a downloadable template to facilitate this.

Clinical vignette: A 25-year-old woman who has been drinking since her teens recently had an episode of binge drinking. During the session, you identify that the trigger was a phone call with her mother, during which the patient felt confronted by the fact that she had recently been fired from her job. The ANT was, "My mother doesn't care about me. She doesn't understand what I'm going through." The emotion was anger. The action was drinking two bottles of white wine over the course of the evening. You intervene to show her that her thoughts about her mother led directly to her anger and drinking, and then help her question the accuracy of those thoughts. She agrees that her mother does, in fact, care about her, and that this more balanced thought would have led her to reach out to her mother for help rather than turning away in anger.

Common ANTs and Other Cognitive Distortions in AUD

- *Permission-giving beliefs:* A patient may think, "I've had a rough day and I haven't had a drink in 30 days. I deserve one drink to relax." Encourage a replacement thought, such as: "I deserve to have another day of sobriety. I know I'll feel bad about myself if I start drinking again."
- *Slip vs relapse:* A slip is a single, isolated use of alcohol after a period of abstinence; a relapse is a prolonged return to a drinking lifestyle. Patients who have a slip may think, "Now I've relapsed. There's nothing I can do about it. It shows how weak I am." Help them understand that slips are common and expected during recovery and do not have to lead to relapse.
- *Cravings:* Cravings can overcome patients. When they are strong, they lead to thoughts like, "There's no way I can live with this feeling. I have to get a drink." Educate that a craving is a temporary physical sensation that will diminish if the patient can find something to take their mind off it for a while (such as calling a sponsor, going to the gym, or eating a nice meal).

Automatic Negative Thought Worksheet for Cognitive Behavioral Therapy

Introduction

A key ingredient of cognitive behavioral therapy (CBT) for alcohol use disorder is discussing automatic negative thoughts that may trigger drinking (see "Cognitive Behavioral Therapy Techniques in Alcohol Use Disorder" for more information). This is a template of a worksheet you can use with your patients to facilitate this technique. Typically, you and your patient would fill out one of these worksheets together during a visit, and then you would ask your patient to do this exercise at least once every week as a homework assignment, and to bring the completed worksheet to the next visit for discussion. This template includes an example from the vignette discussed in the CBT fact sheet. You can download this template and adapt it as needed for your practice setting.

Date	Situation	Automatic Negative Thought	Emotions	Behavior	Rational Positive Response
June 1	Difficult phone call with parent	"She doesn't care about me."	Hopelessness, anger	Drank two bottles of wine	"She does care and wants to help me."

Teaching Relapse Prevention Techniques in Alcohol Use Disorder

Introduction

Relapse rates to alcohol use are approximately 40%–80%, depending on the duration of sobriety. Since relapse is the rule rather than the exception, it is important to make relapse prevention an integral part of treating alcohol use disorder patients. This fact sheet offers some powerful tips and techniques that you can integrate into your treatment visits.

- Start the conversation: "Do you see any barriers that would be a problem to your recovery?" "Is there something that could derail your abstinence?"
- Encourage planning ahead: "What are some situations where you will be tempted to use?"
- Teach refusal skills—strategies for successfully turning down opportunities to drink:
  - Help patients come up with excuses for not drinking other than stating that they have a drinking problem, eg: "My doctor said I shouldn't drink because of heartburn pain." "I find I don't sleep well when I have a drink at night." "I have to stay clear-headed because I have some work I need to do later tonight to prepare for a presentation."
  - Come up with a list of alternative activities to drinking.
  - Suggest use of a non-alcoholic beverage during social functions.
- Teach the HALT mnemonic (Hungry, Angry, Lonely, Tired) as a memory aid for emotional and physical states that can lead to relapse.
- Go over the most common causes of relapse, along with suggestions to deal with each one:
  - Self-medication (drinking to deal with stress): Find other activities to deal with stress.
  - Temptation (responding to triggers): Avoid situations that trigger cravings (such as liquor stores, bars, or parties).
  - Overconfidence that they can drink moderately: Remember that controlled drinking often leads to relapse.
  - Boredom: Take up a new hobby, especially one unrelated to their drinking friends. Get involved in Alcoholics Anonymous (AA) in sponsor or other leadership roles.
- Recommend journaling, which can help to identify situations that might lead to relapse: "Write half a page a day in your journal, and bring your notebook to sessions."
- Help the patient write a recovery plan: a schedule of activities that will help with sobriety, such as AA meetings, regular check-ins with sponsors, and regular involvement in non-drinking activities.
- Encourage the patient to start and end each day by committing to sobriety:
  - "Start the day by reading something focused on recovery and then mindfully planning the day."
  - "End the day by confirming you are following your recovery plan."

Alcoholics Anonymous Meetings: The Basics

Introduction

Research has shown that consistent attendance at Alcoholics Anonymous (AA) meetings is at least as effective as any other treatment, and possibly more so. The two key ingredients of AA meetings are:

- Making positive changes in social networks
- Learning coping skills to maintain abstinence when in high-risk social situations

What Are the 12 Steps?

The essential idea: Stopping alcohol use is only the beginning of a journey. In order to maintain sobriety, alcohol must be replaced with something just as compelling. The 12 steps represent a series of guidelines for how people might choose to live their lives without alcohol.

The steps can be broken down into three phases: Surrendering, Confessing, and Maintaining (memory aid: "SCM"— "AA is no SCAM").

Steps 1–3: Surrendering

- 1: Admit being powerless over alcohol
- 2: Accept that a higher power can restore your sanity (traditional AA steps refer to God as the higher power, but patients may substitute whatever they find appropriate)
- 3: Decide to turn your will over to that higher power

Steps 4–9: Confessing

- 4: Write out a moral inventory of your behaviors due to alcohol use
- 5: Find someone to confess to (eg, a sponsor or therapist: "We are as sick as our secrets")
- 6 and 7: Prepare yourself mentally to make necessary changes in your life
- 8: Make a list of people you have harmed
- 9: Make direct amends to these people

Steps 10–12: Maintaining

- 10: Take a daily personal inventory (eg, take time at the beginning and end of each day to reflect on behaviors)
- 11: Engage in daily prayer/meditation (eg, pray for inner strength to maintain sobriety)
- 12: Help others (eg, become an AA sponsor or help in other ways)

How Do AA Meetings Work?

- Patients can find local meetings by going to the AA website and entering their ZIP code. Research has shown that the threshold for effectiveness is attending at least one meeting per week. Meetings are free.
- There are many categories and flavors of meetings: groups for alcohol use vs polysubstance use, gender-specific or age-specific groups, professional groups, etc. Remind patients: "If you don't like one meeting, try another."
- Meetings last an hour. First-timers will introduce themselves (eg, the new arrival will say, "Hi, my name is Danny and I'm an alcoholic" and members will respond, "Hi Danny"). Meetings might focus on a particular step or have a guest speaker.
- Eventually attendees should find a sponsor. Patients might start by getting together a "phone list," which includes a few people whom they are comfortable with and who are willing to make themselves available to talk.

How to Help Families of Alcohol Users: An Overview

Introduction

Families or friends of patients may ask you for advice about what they can do to help their loved one with alcohol use disorder (AUD). Some will be quite desperate for help, and may themselves be suffering from psychiatric illness—possibly aggravated by the patient's behaviors. In this fact sheet we give you an overview of the different things you can suggest for family members. Some of these options are covered in more detail in individual fact sheets.

- **Family meetings (see "How to Conduct a Family Meeting")**
  - What they are: Informal meetings that you conduct in the office, where you discuss the patient's alcohol use issues and how the family can be helpful
  - Pros:
    - Meetings are easy to implement
    - You can learn more about your patient in a family meeting than in individual sessions
    - You have direct input into the family's involvement with treatment
  - Cons:
    - Meetings can interfere with your therapeutic alliance if the patient perceives that you're taking the family's "side"
    - Things can get heated—you can't predict what family members will say and what their agendas may be

- **Al-Anon/Alateen (see "Al-Anon/Alateen" fact sheet)**
  - What they are: 12-step groups for families/friends of people with AUD
  - Pros:
    - Group meetings are often co-located with other 12-step meetings so the patient and family/friends can attend different meetings at the same time in the same location
    - Loved ones can receive support regardless of whether the patient is interested in quitting drinking
  - Cons:
    - Not everyone resonates with the 12-step model
    - Every individual meeting is a little bit different in terms of group dynamic, so families/friends may need to try various meetings to find a good fit

- **Community reinforcement and family training (CRAFT)**
  - What it is: A therapeutic technique in which a therapist works with the family to optimize the home environment and facilitate sobriety or entry into treatment
  - Pros:
    - Family members obtain tools to facilitate reduction in drinking, such as communication, setting limits, and establishing appropriate consequences
    - Studies have shown that CRAFT is more effective in promoting sobriety than techniques such as 12-step facilitation therapy
  - Cons:
    - Professionals skilled in this technique can be difficult to find

- **Intervention (see "Staging Interventions for Alcohol Use Disorder")**
  - What it is: A family meeting, usually facilitated by a professional interventionist, where the individual with AUD is gently confronted and usually given an ultimatum to encourage them to enter treatment
  - Pros:
    - An intervention makes it clear to the individual that others are very concerned about their drinking
    - The patient may be convinced to undergo rapid entry into a treatment program
  - Cons:
    - An intervention requires significant commitment from attendees (friends, family members, employers, etc.)
    - Attendees must hold at least one rehearsal/planning meeting before the intervention
    - Outcomes are variable—the patient may refuse treatment despite family pressure or ultimatums
    - The interventionist may have a financial incentive to get the patient into a specific residential treatment program

How to Conduct a Family Meeting

Introduction

Including family meetings in your treatment of alcohol-using patients (or any psychiatric patients, for that matter) can help you better understand treatment challenges and therefore help achieve long-term sobriety. But it can be awkward to facilitate such meetings, especially if you haven't done many. This fact sheet presents some useful tips.

Meeting Structure and Planning

- *Decide whom to include.* Usually family meetings work best when they include the patient and one or two very close loved ones, such as a spouse/partner or first-degree relatives. Smaller meetings are more manageable.
- *Obtain permission.* If the meeting does not include the patient, have the patient sign a release of information form that explicitly allows a discussion of alcohol use issues.
- *Introduce the purpose of the meeting.* Say something like, "I think it's important to have this meeting with John and his family to make sure everyone is on the same page and to support John in his recovery."
- *Describe the ground rules.* Stick to the time limit. Keep things respectful—there should be no yelling, insults, blaming, or interrupting. Don't allow anyone to monopolize the conversation. Keep the meeting productive. Emphasize problem-solving, rather than problem-describing.

Meeting Content

- *Help the loved one with matters conducive to recovery.* This can include:
  - Assist with transportation to appointments
  - Support medication adherence (eg, taking disulfiram for alcohol use disorder)
  - Have family meals together as much as possible
  - Support a regular sleep/wake cycle
  - Support alternatives to alcohol, such as alternative activities (exercise, gardening, cooking, crafting, outdoor activities, music, etc.) and alternative beverages
  - Prevent and respond to relapse, such as by identifying typical signs of relapse and discussing the use of technology such as breathalyzers and ignition interlock devices. Remind family members that criticizing and blaming are less helpful than providing support for recovery.
- *Don't help the loved one with matters that are not conducive to recovery.* For example:
  - Don't give them money if they have repeatedly spent it on using
  - Don't use alcohol around them
  - Don't turn a blind eye to obvious red flags of relapse
- *Help the loved one take care of themselves.*
  - If available in your community, recommend support groups such as Al-Anon/Alateen and SMART Recovery Family & Friends
  - Refer meeting attendees to the following online resources:
    - National Institute on Alcohol Abuse and Alcoholism (NIAAA) Alcohol Treatment Navigator (https://alcoholtreatment.niaaa.nih.gov)
    - National Institute on Drug Abuse (NIDA) section for patients and families (https://nida.nih.gov/nidamed-medical-health-professionals/for-your-patients)
    - Substance Abuse and Mental Health Services Administration (SAMHSA) Resources for Families Coping With Mental Health and Substance Use Disorders (https://www.samhsa.gov/families)
  - Recommend the book *Get Your Loved One Sober: Alternatives to Nagging, Pleading, and Threatening* by Robert Meyers and Brenda Wolfe

Al-Anon/Alateen Fact Sheet

Introduction

When family members need support from others who are also struggling with a loved one's substance use issues, referring them to Al-Alon or Alateen is a great option.

What They Are

Al-Anon is a mutual support group for people whose lives are affected by someone else's drinking. It was founded in 1951, and its name was created from the first syllables of its parent organization **Al**coholics **Anon**ymous (AA). Alateen was founded in 1957 as a branch of Al-Anon for teenage relatives and friends of people with alcohol addiction.

How They Work

Like other 12-step groups, Al-Anon and Alateen are non-professional, peer-run fellowships, with meetings led by long-time members. The groups work with the idea that alcoholism is a family illness, but they do not aim to alter the drinking of affected loved ones. Rather, members admit they are powerless over their loved one's drinking and keep the focus on their own well-being by working through the approach's 12 steps. Al-Anon/Alateen help frustrated family members to realize that the drinker's behavior is not their fault. The groups also provide education about how not to enable drinkers, emphasizing that allowing them to experience the consequences of their actions can lead them toward recovery—often described as a "tough love" approach.

Website

https://al-anon.org/for-members/members-resources/literature/feature-publications/

Key Publication

How Al-Anon Works for Families & Friends of Alcoholics

Pros

- Group meetings are free (donations are encouraged but not required) and widely available, with more than 24,000 Al-Anon groups and nearly 1,400 Alateen groups worldwide.
- Online and phone meetings are available.
- Meetings are potentially open to loved ones of people struggling with drug (as well as alcohol) addictions.

Cons

- While Al-Anon/Alateen are effective for emotional support, they are not very effective at encouraging loved ones to enter into treatment for their addictions.
- The Al-Anon/Alateen approach teaches detachment. Members may perceive helpful or necessary actions (such as driving their loved one to the emergency room) as a form of enabling. They may feel that the loved one needs to "hit rock bottom" before they can improve, which can have serious consequences and is not supported by evidence.

Clinical Pearls

- Recommend Al-Anon/Alateen for family members needing emotional support. Recommend community reinforcement and family training (CRAFT) for families wanting to focus more on encouraging loved ones to get into treatment. (See "How to Help Families of Alcohol Users: An Overview" for more on CRAFT.)
- Al-Anon/Alateen meetings are often held at the same time and location as AA meetings—but in a different room— so that family members can attend Al-Anon/Alateen while the person with alcohol use disorder (AUD) attends the AA meeting.
- Adult Children of Alcoholics (ACA; https://adultchildren.org) is another 12-step mutual-help group to keep in mind. ACA's focus is recovering from the aftermath of growing up in a family affected by AUD.

Interesting Fact

When Love Is Not Enough: The Lois Wilson Story (2010) is a film about the early years of AA and Al-Anon, co-founded by Bill W. and his wife Lois W., respectively.

Staging Interventions for Alcohol Use Disorder

Introduction

An intervention is a planned meeting with the patient, the family, and usually an addiction professional (an interventionist). The purpose is to confront a patient reluctant to seek treatment with information from family and friends in the hopes of encouraging treatment seeking.

How It Works

- First there is a pre-intervention meeting among people who are most concerned about the patient—family, friends, an employer, a probation officer, etc. At this meeting, attendees discuss their concerns about the patient, rehearse the statements of concern they intend to make, and schedule the intervention meeting where the patient will be encouraged to engage in treatment.
- The actual intervention is typically a surprise to the patient. At the intervention, people will express their concerns and generally voice an ultimatum that will take effect if the patient refuses treatment. These consequences may include separation, divorce, denial of parental rights, termination of employment, or formal violation of probation, among others.
- The ideal outcome is for the patient to agree to enter treatment immediately, with the interventionist taking them directly to the program from the meeting. The intervention may alternatively aim to get the patient to agree to quit drinking or to enter outpatient treatment.
- Often the interventionist works with one or more residential treatment programs and will get a kickback if the patient enters the program.

Potential Challenges

- Family members may not feel comfortable with direct confrontation or may not be willing to follow through on the consequences.
- The patient may superficially agree to enter treatment but then renege on that commitment after the meeting.

What You Can Do

- Help family members find an interventionist. This is typically done by contacting a local addiction treatment facility.
- Be honest with family members about the need for resolute commitment to the ultimatum for an intervention to be successful.

Bottom Line

In general, we are not big fans of the intervention approach because it is inherently confrontational and requires a sustained level of commitment from family members. It is also hard to find an interventionist who does not have a conflict of interest with a particular residential facility.

How to Choose the Right Medications for Alcohol Use Disorder

Introduction

This fact sheet is specifically for long-term medication treatment to decrease use and to prevent relapse. See the individual medication fact sheets for details on each first- and second-line medication listed here. Other fact sheets focus on medications for alcohol withdrawal.

First-Line Treatments

Naltrexone (ReVia [oral pill], Vivitrol [monthly injection])

- *Mechanism of action:* Blocks opioid receptors, reducing the rewarding effect of drinking.
- *Key points:* Usual dose 50 mg daily. First choice for most patients. Well tolerated (main side effect is transient nausea), can be taken as a single daily pill, and can be started while actively drinking. Also available as a once-monthly injection (Vivitrol); this is especially good for patients with adherence issues, for whom the injection is recommended as first line over the oral tablets. Can be combined with other alcohol use disorder meds and is especially effective when combined with gabapentin.

Acamprosate (Campral)

- *Mechanism of action:* Unclear; may enhance GABA activity.
- *Key points:* Dose is 666 mg three times a day. Second choice after naltrexone. Best for patients who have already achieved abstinence and for patients with liver disease (it does not require hepatic metabolism). Its effect on GABA reduces anxiety in some. Drawbacks: Less compelling efficacy evidence; must take two large pills three times a day.

Second-Line Treatments

Gabapentin (Gralise, Horizant, Neurontin)

- *Mechanism of action:* Unclear; may blunt neuronal hyperexcitability by boosting central GABA.
- *Key points:* Higher dose (1800 mg daily) works better than 900 mg daily. Can be combined with naltrexone, and it augmented the efficacy of naltrexone in one trial. Good for patients with liver disease (it does not require hepatic metabolism). Can also be helpful for patients who have anxiety symptoms. If it is used to manage mild alcohol withdrawal syndrome, then it can be continued for long-term treatment of alcohol use disorder. Drawbacks: Can cause sedation; can be misused for recreational effect; risky in patients with opioid use disorder.

Topiramate (Eprontia, Qudexy XR, Topamax, Trokendi XR)

- *Mechanism of action:* Blocks glutamate, which in turn reduces dopamine, dampening alcohol's reinforcing effect.
- *Key points:* Shown to reduce the number of heavy drinking days. To mitigate side effects, titrate slowly up to 100–150 mg BID over six to eight weeks. Often used at bedtime to minimize side effects. Drawbacks: Cognitive slowing.

Disulfiram (Antabuse)

- *Mechanism of action:* Dosed from 250 mg to 500 mg daily. Creates a buildup of acetaldehyde by inhibiting aldehyde dehydrogenase, causing very uncomfortable flushing, headache, tachycardia, nausea, and vomiting if patient consumes alcohol. Disulfiram is an aversive treatment and does not decrease cravings.
- *Key points:* Best for patients who are abstinent, are highly motivated to remain sober, and have caretakers directly observing adherence. Drawbacks: Impulsive patients may drink on disulfiram and risk a reaction; can cause metallic taste; may worsen psychotic symptoms; not good for patients with cardiac disease due to the stress of the alcohol reaction and similarity to heart attack symptoms.

Treatments to Consider When Nothing Else Works

Varenicline (Chantix)

- *Mechanism of action:* Nicotine receptor partial agonist.
- *Key points:* May decrease cravings. Best for patients who smoke and drink; may be more effective in men than women.

Ondansetron (Zofran)

- *Mechanism of action:* 5HT-3 antagonist.
- *Key points:* Works best in those who started drinking at a young age.

Alcohol Withdrawal Management

Alcohol Withdrawal Time Course and Symptoms

Time Course

- Alcohol withdrawal symptom onset: Usually within six to eight hours of last drink, though in some very heavy drinkers, withdrawal may not begin until 24 hours after last drink.
- Peak withdrawal: Within 24–48 hours.
- Duration of withdrawal:
  - Mild withdrawal will usually last not more than 72 hours (three days) after symptoms begin.
  - More severe withdrawal can last significantly longer and involve the symptoms below.

Symptoms

- Initial symptoms: Insomnia, anxiety, tremor, sweating, palpitations, headache, gastrointestinal upset.
- Progressive symptoms: Nausea, irritability, elevated blood pressure, tachycardia, elevated body temperature, diaphoresis, increased tremulousness, hyperarousal, and disorientation.
- Withdrawal seizures typically occur within six to 48 hours after last drink and present as generalized, tonic-clonic seizures with a short postictal period.
  - A history of withdrawal seizures increases risk of subsequent seizures (kindling effect).
  - Untreated seizures can progress to delirium tremens (DT) in one-third of patients.
- Alcoholic hallucinosis involves hallucinations that develop within 12–48 hours after last drink and occur with clear sensorium and minimal vital sign changes.
  - Are usually visual, though can occur in any sensory modality.
  - Can persist for up to one week after last drink.
- DT is the most severe form of alcohol withdrawal. It presents with disorientation, hallucinations or illusions, tremors, tachycardia, hypertension, hyperthermia, anxiety, agitation, and diaphoresis.
  - Usually begins 48–96 hours after last drink and can last up to two weeks.
  - DT is a life-threatening condition with mortality ranges of 5%–8%. Death most commonly occurs due to arrhythmias or complications from comorbid medical conditions.

How to Predict Severity of Alcohol Withdrawal

Introduction

Predicting the severity of withdrawal is important for deciding on the right treatment setting. Will your patient need inpatient treatment, or will outpatient treatment be sufficient? And if inpatient is needed, will they need to be treated in the ICU, or will a psychiatric unit suffice? In this fact sheet, we help you predict the severity of withdrawal in a given patient.

Predictive of Less Severe Withdrawal

- Patient reports only minimal symptoms of withdrawal in the past (eg, they felt sweaty and shaky but those symptoms went away on their own within days)
- Binge drinking pattern (eg, weekend drinkers); such patients rarely experience withdrawal symptoms, because they are used to the rapid rise and fall in blood alcohol level (BAL), so they don't establish the same tolerance as daily drinkers

Predictive of More Severe Withdrawal

- Long duration of heavy and regular alcohol use
- Early signs of withdrawal even though the patient has a positive BAL—this indicates that they drink so continuously that they are unable to tolerate a low BAL
- Marked autonomic hyperactivity on presentation (eg, elevated systolic BP on presentation, pulse >100 bpm)
- Comorbid medical illness (especially coronary artery disease and alcohol-related liver disease)
- Older age (>65 years)
- Physiologic dependence on benzodiazepines in addition to alcohol use
- The following lab abnormalities have been correlated with more severe withdrawal:
  - Serum chloride <96 mmol/L (this is the main "inhibiting" ion in the CNS, so a low level indicates hyperexcitability)
  - Low platelet count
  - Low hemoglobin (anemia)
  - High alanine transaminase (ALT)

Scales to Predict Severity of Alcohol Withdrawal

- PAWSS (Prediction of Alcohol Withdrawal Severity Scale)
  - 10-item scale
  - 100% specificity and sensitivity in predicting moderate to severe withdrawal
  - Ref: Maldonado JR et al, *Alcohol* 2014;48(4):375–390
- LARS (Luebeck Alcohol Withdrawal Risk Scale)
  - 11-item shortened version
  - Specifically designed to predict severe alcohol withdrawal syndrome (AWS) among patients without significant comorbid illness
    - Prospective study of 100 patients in a hospital psychiatric unit
  - 100% sensitivity and 88% specificity to differentiate severe AWS from mild to moderate AWS

How to Manage Alcohol Withdrawal in Outpatient Settings

Criteria for Outpatient Withdrawal

Outpatient managed withdrawal is best for patients who are medically healthy, have no history of seizures, have good psychosocial supports, are reliable (answer phone calls, follow instructions exactly, and return for appointments), and have no major or unstable mental illness.

Clinical Tips

- Inform your patient that they should take time off from work/school and other responsibilities for the initial few days of outpatient withdrawal management
- Your patient should not be alone during treatment of withdrawal—they can stay with a family member, a friend, or an AA sponsor (or the family member/friend can stay with your patient)
- It is often helpful to give the patient a chart or calendar of each day's dosing schedule to avoid confusion and missed or extra doses (see "Medication Tapering Instructions" for a sample you can use)
- The patient must be willing to abort the outpatient protocol and go to the emergency department or an inpatient withdrawal treatment program if you determine that the withdrawal syndrome is worsening and your patient's safety is at risk

Mild Outpatient Withdrawal With Gabapentin

- Prescribe gabapentin 300 mg #30, no refills
- Instruct patient to take one pill every six to eight hours as needed for withdrawal symptoms
- Check in with patient in two to three days to assess; if symptoms are more severe, may need to add benzodiazepines
- Gabapentin is advantageous for withdrawal because (unlike benzos) it can be continued for long-term treatment to prevent future alcohol relapse

Moderate Outpatient Withdrawal With Benzodiazepines

Clonazepam (Klonopin) is usually the first-choice benzodiazepine for outpatient withdrawal due to a lower likelihood of causing euphoria. Use a tapering protocol of five to 10 days as detailed below.

- Prescribe clonazepam 0.5 mg #30, no refills
- Days 1–2: Start with 1 mg QID (may have to decrease initial dose depending on sedation—give patient instructions and latitude to adjust dose if needed)
- Day 3: Start gradual taper by one 0.5 mg pill per day, depending on patient tolerability
- Days 4–10: Gradual taper and discontinuation

You can also use any other benzodiazepine for outpatient withdrawal; see below for recommendations on initial prescription and initial dosing. All will be tapered gradually, similar to the protocol for clonazepam.

- Chlordiazepoxide (Librium): Initial script 25 mg #30; initial dose 50 mg QID
- Diazepam (Valium): Initial script 10 mg #30; initial dose 20 mg QID
- Oxazepam (Serax): Initial script 15 mg #30; initial dose 30 mg QID
- Lorazepam (Ativan): Initial script 0.5 mg #30; initial dose 1 mg QID
- Phenobarbital (see "How to Use Phenobarbital to Manage Alcohol Withdrawal" for details)

How to Manage Alcohol Withdrawal in Inpatient Settings

Criteria for Inpatient Detox

Inpatient managed withdrawal is best for patients with significant consistent alcohol use daily for months, history of seizures, significant medical issues, severe concurrent mental illness, and unstable home environment/poor outpatient reliability (see "How to Predict Severity of Alcohol Withdrawal").

Symptom-Triggered Withdrawal Protocol (CIWA Protocol)

Symptom-triggered protocols are the most commonly used method for inpatient managed withdrawal. In this method you use a scale to measure withdrawal symptoms, and then you dose medications based on the severity of the symptoms.

Symptom-triggered protocols have a number of advantages that make them popular: They allow flexibility in increasing or decreasing benzo dosing based on real-time patient need; they are safer in severe withdrawal when you may need to use very high benzo doses to prevent complications like seizures; and they allow for shorter admissions for patients with less severe withdrawal. Disadvantage: Patients may become adept at faking or exaggerating withdrawal symptoms to get more benzos.

- Clinical Institute Withdrawal Scale (CIWA) assessment on admission and every two to six hours depending on severity of symptoms
- Initial loading dose of benzo given on admission (eg, Librium 50 mg or Valium 20 mg PO; or Serax 30 mg or Ativan 1 mg for those with liver disease)
- Sliding scale given based on CIWA scores:
  - 0–4: Absence of withdrawal, no medication
  - 5–11: Mild withdrawal, Librium 25 mg or Serax 15 mg
  - 12–20: Moderate withdrawal, Librium 50 mg or Serax 30 mg
  - >20: Severe withdrawal, Librium 75 mg or Serax 45 mg
- CIWA discontinued when patient scores below 5 for 24 hours
- Typical detox lasts three to four days

Scheduled Dosing

In some cases, inpatients will do better with scheduled tapers. This is especially true for patients who appear to be amplifying their symptoms to obtain more medications, or who have underlying anxiety disorders leading them to request benzos to treat anxiety as opposed to withdrawal.

Here is a typical scheduled dose protocol using Librium (five-day protocol; can be shorter if withdrawal symptoms are milder):

- Loading dose of Librium 50 mg on admission (or Valium 20 mg, Serax 30 mg, Ativan 1 mg depending on preference and patient characteristics)
- Day 1: Librium 50 mg QID
- Days 2 and 3: Librium 50 mg PO TID
- Day 4: Librium 50 mg PO BID
- Day 5: Librium 50 mg PO at bedtime (last day of Librium)

Hybrid Management (Scheduled Plus CIWA)

Start on scheduled dosing but order CIWA assessments in addition. This allows staff to increase the benzodiazepine dose if the CIWA is high, or to decrease the dose if the patient seems oversedated.

Comfort Medications

Many psychiatric hospitals have a list of standard as-needed comfort meds that are sometimes added to manage symptoms of withdrawal. In general, we discourage their use, because if your patient is reporting breakthrough withdrawal symptoms of anxiety, jitteriness, insomnia, etc., the better solution is to increase the dose of the benzodiazepine. However, if you choose to supplement benzos with other agents, here is a reasonable menu of choices.

- For anxiety:
  - Clonidine 0.1 mg PO Q6 hours as needed; hold for systolic blood pressure <90 or heart rate <60
  - Hydroxyzine 25–50 mg Q6 hours as needed
- For insomnia:
  - Trazodone 50 mg PO QHS as needed
- For nausea:
  - Ondansetron 4 mg PO or IM Q8 hours as needed

How to Choose a Benzodiazepine for Alcohol Withdrawal

Introduction

There are many benzodiazepines to choose from. Generally they are all effective for alcohol withdrawal, and the key thing is to pick one that you are comfortable with and get familiar with its use. Nonetheless, some benzos have become favorites of addiction specialists, and in this sheet we provide some guidelines for how to decide on benzos for specific patients.

Patients Without Significant Liver Disease

Chlordiazepoxide (Librium)

- *Advantages:* Long acting; active metabolites, allowing for smoother detox with fewer breakthrough withdrawal symptoms between doses
- *Disadvantages:* More euphoria, so patient may be more likely to request extra doses; not available as injectable

Diazepam (Valium)

- *Advantages:* Long acting; active metabolites, allowing for smoother detox with fewer breakthrough withdrawal symptoms between doses; available as injectable
- *Disadvantages:* More euphoria, so patient may be more likely to request extra doses

Clonazepam (Klonopin)

- *Advantages:* Long acting; active metabolites, allowing for smoother detox with fewer breakthrough withdrawal symptoms between doses; less euphoria than the others
- *Disadvantages:* Not available as injectable

Patients With Significant Liver Disease

By "significant" liver disease, we mean disease severe enough to interfere with metabolism of medications. This is limited to patients with cirrhosis or symptomatic alcoholic hepatitis. Patients presenting with asymptomatic transaminitis with normal bilirubin and albumin can generally metabolize meds normally and can tolerate long-acting benzodiazepines.

Oxazepam (Serax)

- *Advantages:* Short acting; no active metabolites; won't build up in liver disease
- *Disadvantages:* Breakthrough withdrawal symptoms more prevalent; not available as injectable

Lorazepam (Ativan)

- *Advantages:* Intermediate acting; no active metabolites; oral tablet can be given sublingually or rectally if necessary; available as injectable
- *Disadvantages:* Breakthrough withdrawal symptoms prevalent, though not as prevalent as with oxazepam

Phenobarbital

- *Advantages:* Long acting; less euphoria; safe in liver disease because one-third is excreted unchanged
- *Disadvantages:* Because it is ultra long acting (100-hour half-life), patients can become sedated if given too much too quickly

How to Use Phenobarbital to Manage Alcohol Withdrawal

Introduction

Phenobarbital is becoming more popular as a strategy for managing alcohol withdrawal syndrome (AWS) as clinicians gain more experience with it. A recent retrospective study compared phenobarbital with lorazepam for AWS and found that patients using phenobarbital had a shorter length of stay (2.8 vs 3.6 days) as well as fewer readmissions and emergency room visits after discharge (Hawa F et al, *Cureus* 2021;13(2):e13282).

Special Qualities of Phenobarbital

- Less addictive than benzodiazepines (due to more gradual onset, it is less likely to cause euphoria)
- Less commonly prescribed, so less likely for patients to obtain extra doses via diversion
- Safer in patients with liver damage, due to:
  - Less dependence on liver metabolism (one-third excreted unchanged)
  - No active metabolites, so no metabolite buildup in liver disease
- Longest half-life of any sedative, about 100 hours; allows less frequent dosing and often no need for tapering due to gradual metabolism

Phenobarbital Protocol for Outpatient Detox

- Prescribe phenobarbital 15 mg, 30 pills, no refills
- Day 1: Start with loading dose: 30 mg PO Q6 hours; tell patient they can take an extra dose between scheduled doses if they feel shaky or sweaty
- Day 2: See patient (telehealth or in-person visit) to assess if loading dose was sufficient to prevent withdrawal symptoms; adjust upward or downward as needed
- Day 3: Instruct patient to gradually taper phenobarbital over the next eight days (for 10 days of detox total), typically by one pill per day, usually by decreasing daytime doses before nighttime doses
- Days 4–10: See chart below for more specific instructions (in this example, the loading dose is 30 mg Q6 hours); most patients do best with such clear guidance

Outpatient Alcohol Detox Regimen With Phenobarbital

	Day 1	Day 2	Day 3	Day 4	Day 5	Day 6	Day 7	Day 8	Day 9	Day 10
6 am	15, 15	15, 15	15, 15	15, 15	15	15	15 three times daily	15 twice daily	15 once daily	15 once every few days until discontinuation
12 pm	15, 15	15, 15	15	15	15	15				
6 pm	15, 15	15, 15	15, 15	15	15	15				
12 am	15, 15	15, 15	15, 15	15, 15	15, 15	15				

Notes: "15" refers to 15 mg phenobarbital. "Day 1" etc. are illustrative and may need adjusting in patients who cannot tolerate this taper rate.

Phenobarbital Hybrid Protocol for Inpatient Detox

The hybrid protocol is similar to the outpatient protocol, but you can shorten to a four-day taper and start with higher doses. Prescribe standing doses but also evaluate symptoms with CIWA; instruct the patient to decrease dose if they are experiencing sedation, or increase dose if they are having significant withdrawal symptoms.

- Days 1 and 2: 60 mg Q6 hours (with upward or downward adjustments based on CIWA assessments)
- Day 3: 30 mg/15 mg/15 mg/30 mg (Q6 hour administration)
- Day 4: 15 mg Q6 hours
- Day 5: Stop
- Note: Most patients can be more rapidly treated by taking a loading dose of 60 mg Q6 hours for one day, then stopping; phenobarbital's long half-life means that usually no tapering is needed

Medication Tapering Instructions

Introduction

Regardless of which withdrawal regimen you choose, if your patient doesn't understand the schedule of administration, they are unlikely to be successful. This fact sheet consists of a basic template of a tapering schedule that clarifies exactly how many pills they should take when.

Patient Name: _____

Date: _____

Name of Medication: _____

Dose Strength: _____

Day of Week	Date	Number of Pills to Take for Each Dose			
		Time of Day	Time of Day	Time of Day	Time of Day

Date of Next Appointment: _____

Clinical Institute Withdrawal Assessment for Alcohol Scale, Revised (CIWA-Ar)

Introduction

The Clinical Institute Withdrawal Assessment for Alcohol Scale, Revised (CIWA-Ar) is the most widely used alcohol withdrawal symptom scale. Although it is primarily used in inpatient settings, it's also useful for outpatient detox since it reminds both clinicians and patients of the types and severity of symptoms seen in alcohol withdrawal.

Patient: _____

Date: _____ Time: _____ (24 hour clock, midnight = 00:00)

Pulse or heart rate, taken for one minute: _____

Blood pressure: _____

NAUSEA AND VOMITING — Ask "Do you feel sick to your stomach? Have you vomited?" Observation.

0   no nausea and no vomiting
1   mild nausea with no vomiting
2
3
4   intermittent nausea with dry heaves
5
6
7   constant nausea, frequent dry heaves and vomiting

TACTILE DISTURBANCES — Ask "Have you any itching, pins and needles sensations, any burning, any numbness, or do you feel bugs crawling on or under your skin?" Observation.

0   none
1   very mild itching, pins and needles, burning or numbness
2   mild itching, pins and needles, burning or numbness
3   moderate itching, pins and needles, burning or numbness
4   moderately severe hallucinations
5   severe hallucinations
6   extremely severe hallucinations
7   continuous hallucinations

TREMOR — Arms extended and fingers spread apart. Observation.

0   no tremor
1   not visible, but can be felt fingertip to fingertip
2
3
4   moderate, with patient's arms extended
5
6
7   severe, even with arms not extended

AUDITORY DISTURBANCES — Ask "Are you more aware of sounds around you? Are they harsh? Do they frighten you? Are you hearing anything that is disturbing to you? Are you hearing things you know are not there?" Observation.

0   not present
1   very mild harshness or ability to frighten
2   mild harshness or ability to frighten
3   moderate harshness or ability to frighten
4   moderately severe hallucinations
5   severe hallucinations

6   extremely severe hallucinations

7   continuous hallucinations

PAROXYSMAL SWEATS — Observation.

0   no sweat visible

1   barely perceptible sweating, palms moist

2

3

4   beads of sweat obvious on forehead

5

6

7   drenching sweats

VISUAL DISTURBANCES — Ask "Does the light appear to be too bright? Is its color different? Does it hurt your eyes? Are you seeing anything that is disturbing to you? Are you seeing things you know are not there?" Observation.

0   not present

1   very mild sensitivity

2   mild sensitivity

3   moderate sensitivity

4   moderately severe hallucinations

5   severe hallucinations

6   extremely severe hallucinations

7   continuous hallucinations

ANXIETY — Ask "Do you feel nervous?" Observation.

0   no anxiety, at ease

1   mild anxious

2

3

4   moderately anxious, or guarded, so anxiety is inferred

5

6

7   equivalent to acute panic states as seen in severe delirium or acute schizophrenic reactions

HEADACHE, FULLNESS IN HEAD — Ask "Does your head feel different? Does it feel like there is a band around your head?" Do not rate for dizziness or lightheadedness. Otherwise, rate severity.

0   not present

1   very mild

2   mild

3   moderate

4   moderately severe

5   severe

6   very severe

7   extremely severe

ORIENTATION AND CLOUDING OF SENSORIUM — Ask "What day is this? Where are you? Who am I?"

0   oriented and can do serial additions

1   cannot do serial additions or is uncertain about date

2   disoriented for date by no more than 2 calendar days

3   disoriented for date by more than 2 calendar days

4   disoriented for place/or person

AGITATION — Observation.

0   normal activity

1   somewhat more than normal activity

2

3

4   moderately fidgety and restless

5

6

7   paces back and forth during most of the interview, or constantly thrashes about

Total **CIWA-Ar** Score _____

_____ Rater's Initials

Maximum Possible Score 67

The **CIWA-Ar** is not copyrighted and may be reproduced freely. This assessment for monitoring withdrawal symptoms requires approximately 5 minutes to administer. The maximum score is 67 (see instrument). Patients scoring less than 10 do not usually need additional medication for withdrawal.

Sullivan JT, Sykora K, Schneiderman J, Naranjo CA, Sellers EM. Assessment of alcohol withdrawal: The revised Clinical Institute Withdrawal Assessment for Alcohol scale (**CIWA-Ar**). *British Journal of Addiction* 84:1353–1357, 1989.

Alcohol Use Disorder Medication Fact Sheets

ACAMPROSATE (Campral) Fact Sheet [G]

Bottom Line

Acamprosate is best for maintaining abstinence in patients who have already quit drinking, but it can be helpful even after patients relapse. Naltrexone is the better choice for patients who are still drinking, since it is better at helping patients quit. Acamprosate is preferred over naltrexone in patients with hepatic impairment.

FDA Indications

Alcohol use disorder.

Dosage Forms

Delayed-release tablets [G]: 333 mg.

Dosage Guidance

- Start 666 mg TID. Give 333 mg TID in patients with renal impairment.
- Can give 999 mg twice a day if patients can't remember to take it three times daily.

Monitoring: No routine monitoring recommended unless clinical picture warrants.

Cost: $$

Side Effects

- Most common: Diarrhea (dose related, transient), weakness, peripheral edema, insomnia, anxiety.
- Serious but rare: Acute renal failure reported in a few cases; suicidal ideation, attempts, and completions rare but greater than with placebo in studies.

Mechanism, Pharmacokinetics, and Drug Interactions

- Mechanism of action is not fully defined; it appears to work by promoting a balance between the excitatory and inhibitory neurotransmitters, glutamate and GABA, respectively (glutamate and GABA activities appear to be disrupted in alcohol dependence). Basically, we don't know how it works—it just does.
- Not metabolized, cleared as unchanged drug by kidneys; t ½: 20–33 hours.
- No significant drug interactions.

Clinical Pearls

- Approved by the FDA in 2004, but it has been used in France and other countries since 1989.
- Does not eliminate or treat symptoms of alcohol withdrawal. Usually prescribed for maintenance of abstinence; may continue even if patient relapses with alcohol.
- Clinically, acamprosate has demonstrated efficacy in more than 25 placebo-controlled trials, and it has generally been found to be more effective than placebo in reducing risk of returning to any drinking and increasing the cumulative duration of abstinence. However, in reducing heavy drinking, acamprosate appears to be no better than placebo.
- Acamprosate can be used with naltrexone or disulfiram (different mechanism of action), although the combination with naltrexone may not increase efficacy per available studies.
- Taking with food is not necessary, but telling patients to take it three times daily with meals as a memory aid may help with compliance.
- Compared to naltrexone and disulfiram, acamprosate is unique in that it is not metabolized by the liver and is not impacted by alcohol use, so it can be administered to patients with hepatitis or liver disease and to patients who continue drinking alcohol.

Fun Fact

The strange dosing of 333 mg is due to the fact that each tablet contains 300 mg of acamprosate and 33 mg of elemental calcium (because it is available as acamprosate calcium salt).

DISULFIRAM (Antabuse) Fact Sheet [G]

Bottom Line

Disulfiram is an aversive treatment, causing a buildup of ethanol's metabolite acetaldehyde in the serum, which in turn causes symptoms such as flushing, dizziness, nausea, and vomiting if patient consumes alcohol. Since disulfiram does not reduce cravings and any alcohol ingestion could result in a reaction, noncompliance can be common. Its use should be reserved for selective, highly motivated patients in conjunction with supportive and psychotherapeutic treatment.

FDA Indications

Alcohol use disorder.

Dosage Forms

Tablets (Antabuse, [G]): 250 mg, 500 mg.

Dosage Guidance

Start 125 mg QPM (must be abstinent from alcohol >12 hours); increase to 250 mg QPM after several days. Some patients find they can drink alcohol without much reaction on the 250 mg dose, so they may need to increase to 500 mg/day.

Monitoring: Liver function tests if liver disease is suspected.

Cost: $

Side Effects

- Most common: Skin eruptions (eg, acne, allergic dermatitis), drowsiness, fatigue, impotence, headache, metallic taste.
- Serious but rare: Severe (very rarely fatal) hepatitis or hepatic failure reported and may occur in patients with or without prior history of abnormal hepatic function. Rare psychotic episodes have been reported. Rarely may cause peripheral neuropathy or optic neuritis.

Mechanism, Pharmacokinetics, and Drug Interactions

- Aldehyde dehydrogenase inhibitor.
- Metabolized primarily through CYP450; t ½ is not defined, but elimination from body is slow, and effects may persist for one or two weeks after last dose.
- While taking disulfiram, and for one to two weeks after stopping, avoid concomitant use of any medications containing alcohol (including topicals) or "disguised" forms of ethanol (cough syrup, some mouthwashes, oral solutions or liquid concentrates containing alcohol such as sertraline). Any medicinal solution labelled as an "elixir" is dissolved in alcohol and must be avoided. Avoid vinegars, cider, extracts, and foods containing ethanol.
- Some medications can cause a disulfiram-like reaction with alcohol, including metronidazole and sulfonylurea diabetic medications such as chlorpropamide and tolbutamide.

Clinical Pearls

- Disulfiram inhibits the enzyme aldehyde dehydrogenase; when taken with alcohol, acetaldehyde levels are increased by five- to 10-fold, causing unpleasant symptoms that include flushing, nausea, vomiting, palpitations, chest pain, vertigo, hypotension, and (in rare instances) cardiovascular collapse and death. These symptoms are the basis for its use as aversion therapy. Common advice to patients: "You'll wish you were dead, but it likely won't kill you."
- Reaction may last from 30–60 minutes to several hours or as long as alcohol remains in the bloodstream.
- Advise patients to carry an identification card or a medical alert bracelet that states they are taking the medication and lists the symptoms of the reaction and clinician contact information.
- Therapy lasts until the patient is fully recovered and a basis for permanent self-control has been established; maintenance therapy may be required for months or even years.

Fun Fact

Disulfiram's anti-protozoal activity may be effective in *Giardia* and *Trichomonas* infections.

GABAPENTIN (Gralise, Horizant, Neurontin) Fact Sheet [G]

Bottom Line
Gabapentin is effective as an off-label medication to ease alcohol withdrawal symptoms and to reduce cravings over the long term in patients with alcohol use disorder (AUD). Just be aware that, like benzodiazepines, gabapentin is often misused and diverted for its euphoriant effect.

FDA Indications
Partial seizures (Neurontin); post-herpetic neuralgia (Gralise, Neurontin); restless legs syndrome (Horizant).

Off-Label Uses
Anxiety disorders; withdrawal from alcohol or benzodiazepines; AUD.

Dosage Forms
- **Capsules (G):** 100 mg, 300 mg, 400 mg.
- **Tablets (G):** 600 mg, 800 mg.
- **Oral solution (G):** 50 mg/mL.
- **ER tablets (Gralise):** 300 mg, 600 mg.
- **ER tablets (Horizant):** 300 mg, 600 mg (gabapentin enacarbil, a prodrug with better bioavailability).

Dosage Guidance
- For AUD (off-label use), start 300 mg QHS and ↑ to 300 mg BID on the second day, then 300 mg TID on the third day. Increase by 300 mg/day increments every few days to a target dose of 1200–1800 mg/day divided TID. If needed, you can increase as high as 3600 mg daily.

Monitoring: No routine monitoring recommended unless clinical picture warrants.

Cost: IR: $; ER: $$$$$

Side Effects
- Most common: Dizziness, somnolence, ataxia, weight gain, dependence.
- Serious but rare: Potentially serious, sometimes fatal multiorgan hypersensitivity (also known as drug reaction with eosinophilia and systemic symptoms, or DRESS); respiratory depression, especially in combination with opioids.

Mechanism, Pharmacokinetics, and Drug Interactions
- Blocks voltage-dependent calcium channels and modulates excitatory neurotransmitter release.
- Not metabolized; excreted unchanged by kidneys; t ½: 5–7 hours.
- Few significant drug interactions, although you may see additive sedative effects with other sedating drugs. Analgesic control may be affected when gabapentin is added to opiates, including decreased levels of hydrocodone (Vicodin) or increased levels of morphine.

Clinical Pearls
- A meta-analysis that pooled results of 10 studies of gabapentin in alcohol withdrawal found it to be at least moderately effective for reducing cravings and managing withdrawal symptoms (Ahmed S et al, *Prim Care Companion CNS Disord* 2019;21(4):19r02465).
- Higher doses of gabapentin seem to be more effective in AUD. One study showed a clear benefit with 1800 mg/day compared to 900 mg/day (Mason BJ et al, *JAMA Intern Med* 2014;174(1):70–77).
- Recreational use and misuse in the general population is also increasing and seems to occur more often with pregabalin than gabapentin, often at supratherapeutic dosing for the euphoric effects. Those with opioid use disorder have much higher gabapentin and pregabalin misuse rates.

NALTREXONE (ReVia, Vivitrol) Fact Sheet [G]

Bottom Line

Naltrexone, an opioid antagonist, is the first-line medication for alcohol use disorder (AUD)—though it is also approved for opioid use disorder (OUD). By reducing the endorphin-mediated euphoria of drinking, it helps people moderate, preventing that first drink from leading to several more. Avoid naltrexone in patients with hepatic impairment or those taking opioid-based pain medications. For OUD, methadone and buprenorphine are more effective for most patients, although naltrexone may be appropriate for highly motivated OUD patients, with injectable preferred over oral.

FDA Indications

Alcohol use disorder; opioid use disorder (relapse prevention following detox).

Off-Label Uses

Self-injurious behavior; gambling disorder.

Dosage Forms

- **Tablets (ReVia, [G]):** 50 mg (scored).
- **Long-acting injection (Vivitrol):** 380 mg.

Dosage Guidance

- AUD: Start at 25 mg QD and increase to 50 mg QD after one or two days if there are no side effects. Can increase to 75 mg QD if no response after four weeks, then to 100 mg QD if needed.
- Injection: 380 mg IM (gluteal) Q4 weeks (for AUD or OUD). Do not initiate therapy until patient is opioid free for at least seven to 10 days (by urinalysis).

Monitoring: Liver function tests before starting treatment if liver disease is suspected; may prescribe safely in presence of mild to moderate elevations, but not if there is acute hepatitis or hepatic failure.

Cost: Tablet: $; injection: $$$$$

Side Effects

- Most common: Headache, nausea, somnolence, vomiting.
- Serious but rare: Black box warning regarding dose-related hepatocellular injury; the difference between safe and hepatotoxic doses appears to be ≤5-fold (narrow therapeutic window). Discontinue if signs/symptoms of acute hepatitis develop.

Mechanism, Pharmacokinetics, and Drug Interactions

- Opioid antagonist.
- Metabolized primarily through non-CYP450 pathway; t ½: 4 hours (5–10 days for IM).
- No significant interactions other than avoiding use with opiates (see below).

Clinical Pearls

- If your patient has tried oral naltrexone for a few months with no clear benefit, consider switching to injectable naltrexone, due to the lack of compliance concerns and steady serum levels.
- Some patients on Vivitrol may benefit from oral naltrexone as a backup, especially toward the end of the four weeks just before the next injection; they may take oral naltrexone 50 mg as needed for cravings while waiting for the next shot.
- In naltrexone-treated patients requiring emergency pain management, consider alternatives to opioids (eg, regional analgesia, non-opioid analgesics, general anesthesia). If opioid therapy is required, patients should be under the direct care of a trained anesthesia provider.

Fun Fact

Methylnaltrexone, a closely related drug, is marketed as Relistor for the treatment of opioid-induced constipation.

TOPIRAMATE (Eprontia, Qudexy XR, Topamax, Trokendi XR) Fact Sheet [G]

Bottom Line

Topiramate is a reasonable off-label choice for alcohol use disorder (AUD) and for antipsychotic-induced weight gain.

FDA Indications

Seizure disorders for patients ≥2 years; migraine prophylaxis.

Off-Label Uses

Alcohol use disorder; bipolar disorder; PTSD; binge-eating disorder; obesity.

Dosage Forms
- **Tablets (G):** 25 mg, 50 mg, 100 mg, 200 mg.
- **Capsules (G):** 15 mg, 25 mg.
- **ER Capsules (Trokendi XR, Qudexy XR, [G]):** 25 mg, 50 mg, 100 mg, 150 mg, 200 mg.
- **Oral solution (Eprontia):** 25 mg/mL.

Dosage Guidance
- AUD (off-label use): Start 25 mg QHS and ↑ by 25 mg/day in weekly increments. Target dose is around 300 mg/day divided BID, but you may have to use a lower dose depending on side effects. The slower the titration (over six to eight weeks recommended), the less chance of the patient noting cognitive slowing.
- Dose timing: Can be given all at HS (especially the ER versions) or split up twice daily.

Monitoring: Baseline and periodic serum bicarbonate.

Cost: IR: $; ER: $$$

Side Effects
- Most common: Somnolence, dizziness, nervousness, ataxia, speech problems, memory difficulties, confusion, anorexia.
- Serious but rare: Decreases in serum bicarbonate (metabolic acidosis) relatively common but usually mild to moderate; more severe cases, including marked reductions to <17 mEq/L, may occur more rarely. Watch for kidney stones, osteomalacia, and acute closed-angle glaucoma (may manifest as changes in color vision).

Mechanism, Pharmacokinetics, and Drug Interactions
- Sodium channel blocker.
- Not metabolized, excreted primarily unchanged; t ½: 21 hours (56 hours for XR); mild CYP3A4 inducer.
- Avoid concomitant use with hydrochlorothiazide, which can increase risk for hypokalemia; monitor potassium. Avoid in patients with metabolic acidosis taking concomitant metformin. Additive effects with sedatives or alcohol. Concurrent use with valproic acid may increase risk of hyperammonemia and associated encephalopathy. Higher doses (>200 mg/day) may decrease levels of some drugs, including contraceptives (CYP450 induction).

Clinical Pearls
- Many published articles have shown some efficacy in a wide range of disorders, including bipolar disorder, PTSD, AUD, binge-eating disorder, and obesity.
- Topiramate's most compelling data are for preventing relapse in AUD, although it has also been shown to reduce heavy drinking days in patients who are still drinking (Johnson BA et al, *JAMA* 2007;298(14):1641–1651).
- One large study including 30,000 people found that topiramate was associated with reductions in alcohol use across all patient populations, regardless of the reason it was prescribed. Drinking went down in patients with and without AUD (Kranzler HR et al, *Addiction* 2022;117(11):2826–2836).
- Some patients may lose weight, but this is not common; the greatest decrease in weight seems to occur in heavier patients (>100 kg). When weight loss occurs, it is often not a large effect (mean of 6 kg) nor is it a sustained effect (patients return to pretreatment weight after 12–18 months).

Fun Fact

The dose-related cognitive effects of topiramate have led some to refer to Topamax as "Dopamax."

Patient Handouts

ACAMPROSATE Fact Sheet for Patients

Generic Name: Acamprosate (a-KAM-pro-sate)

Brand Name:

- Campral
  - Delayed-release enteric-coated tablet: 333 mg

What Does It Treat?

Moderate to severe alcohol use disorder.

How Does It Work?

Acamprosate works in the brain to treat alcohol use disorder. Its exact mechanism is not known, but it has been shown to decrease cravings for alcohol. Especially when combined with other types of therapy or support, it can help people to stop using alcohol and prevent relapse.

How Do I Take It?

Acamprosate is usually taken by mouth as two tablets with or without food three times daily.

How Long Will I Take It?

Acamprosate is taken for 12 months and then can be stopped, but its effects on alcohol cravings will last for at least another 12 months.

What if I Miss a Dose?

If you miss a dose of acamprosate, take it as soon as you remember unless it is closer to the time of your next dose. Do not double your next dose.

What Are Possible Side Effects?

- Most common: Diarrhea, weakness, swelling, insomnia, anxiety.
- Rare: Changes in kidney function.

What Else Should I Know?

- Do not cut, crush, or chew acamprosate tablets; they should be swallowed whole.
- You can take acamprosate with or without food, but taking it with meals may help you to remember to take each of the three daily doses.
- If you have kidney problems, you may need to take a lower dose and be monitored with blood tests while taking acamprosate.

DISULFIRAM Fact Sheet for Patients

Generic Name: Disulfiram (dye-SUL-fee-ram)

Brand Name:
- Antabuse
  - Tablet: 250 mg, 500 mg

What Does It Treat?

Moderate to severe alcohol use disorder.

How Does It Work?

Disulfiram blocks the breakdown of alcohol in the body, which leads to a buildup of a toxic compound that can cause a bad reaction in people who drink alcohol while taking the medication. Especially when combined with other types of therapy or support, it can help encourage people to stop using alcohol.

How Do I Take It?

Disulfiram can be taken once daily by mouth with or without food as a tablet. You must not start taking it until at least 12 hours after your last drink of alcohol.

How Long Will I Take It?

Different people take disulfiram for different lengths of time. Continue taking it as long as you and your provider find it helpful.

What if I Miss a Dose?

If you miss a dose of disulfiram, take it as soon as you remember unless it is closer to the time of your next dose. Do not double your next dose.

What Are Possible Side Effects?

- Most common: Headache, metallic taste, skin eruptions like acne, sleepiness.
- Rare: Changes in liver function.

What Else Should I Know?

- Avoid drinking alcohol and ingesting any other forms of alcohol while taking disulfiram and for one to two weeks after stopping the medication. Other forms of alcohol include creams and ointments, cough syrups, mouthwashes, oral liquid medications, vinegars, ciders, and foods containing alcohol (such as rum cakes, chocolates with liquor inside, and various other desserts that may have alcohol).
- If you drink or ingest alcohol while taking disulfiram, you will experience a very unpleasant reaction that can include flushing, dizziness, nausea, vomiting, sweating, heart palpitations, and chest pain. Call your doctor or go to your nearest emergency room if you experience a reaction.
- Let your health care providers know you are taking disulfiram and consider carrying a wallet card or other alert stating you are taking disulfiram.

NALTREXONE Fact Sheet for Patients

Generic Name: Naltrexone (nal-TREKS-own)

Brand Names:
- ReVia
  - Tablet: 50 mg
- Vivitrol
  - Long-acting injection: 380 mg

What Does It Treat?
Moderate to severe alcohol use disorder.

How Does It Work?
Naltrexone blocks opioid receptors in the brain, which can decrease cravings for and rewarding effects of alcohol or opioids. Especially when combined with other types of therapy or support, it can help people to stop using alcohol or opioids and prevent relapse.

How Do I Take It?
Naltrexone can be taken once daily by mouth with or without food as a tablet, or it can be taken as a once-monthly injection into the muscle. Injections are given in a physician's office or pharmacy, not at home.

How Long Will I Take It?
Different people stay on naltrexone for different lengths of time, but usually it's taken for at least six to 12 months. Continue taking it as long as you and your provider find it helpful.

What if I Miss a Dose?
If you miss a dose of oral naltrexone, take it as soon as you remember unless it is closer to the time of your next dose. Do not double your next dose.

What Are Possible Side Effects?
- Most common: Nausea, vomiting, headache, sleepiness. Bruising, swelling, or tenderness at the site of injection with the injectable form.
- Rare: Changes in liver function.

What Else Should I Know?
- If you experience nausea, try taking your naltrexone dose with food. Or, let your prescriber know and they may reduce your dose.
- If you experience pain in your lower back or excessive tiredness, let your prescriber know.
- Avoid taking any opioids while you are taking naltrexone or if you have recently stopped taking naltrexone.
- Let your health care providers know you are taking naltrexone and consider carrying a wallet card or other alert stating that you are taking naltrexone.

Alcohol Use Disorder: Personal Recovery Plan Template

Personal Triggers That Put Me at Risk for Using

(For example: Going home after work to have unstructured time makes me more likely to drink.)

1. _____
2. _____
3. _____

How I Will Address Each Trigger

(For example: Each day after work, I will go to the gym or to an Alcoholics Anonymous [AA] meeting.)

1. _____
2. _____
3. _____

Ways I Will Increase My Self-Care

(For example: I will go for a long walk in my neighborhood three days a week.)

1. _____
2. _____
3. _____

Coping Skills I Will Learn or Improve and How I Will Do This

(For example: I will take a meditation course and will work up to meditating 20 minutes each day.)

1. _____
2. _____
3. _____

My Relapse Prevention Strategies

(For example: If I feel the urge to drink, I will call my AA sponsor instead.)

1. _____
2. _____
3. _____

Additional Commitments to Help Me Stick to My Plan

(For example: I will be clean and sober for my daughter's graduation celebration in June.)

1. _____
2. _____
3. _____

(Adapted from a template provided by American Addiction Centers: https://recovery.org/pro/articles/
developing-your-personal-recovery-plan-template-included/)

Tips for Recovery From Alcohol Use Disorder (Patient Handout)

Introduction

This patient handout includes basic advice to help your patients stay on track with their alcohol abstinence goals. Feel free to download and to tailor it to your own practice or setting.

Share Your Treatment Goals to Keep Yourself Accountable

- List family members/friends to tell:

  _____

- Potential scripts:
  - "I'm planning to cut down on my drinking and would appreciate your support for this."
  - "I promise not to get mad if you share your concerns with me."
  - "This is important for me to do and I need your support to do it."

Create Specific Drinking Reduction Goals

- How much are you currently drinking?

  _____

- Amount of initial reduction:

  _____

  - Eg: One less glass of wine per night, one less shot per night

- Tips for reducing drinking:
  - Choose beer or wine with lower alcohol content
  - Stay hydrated—have one glass of water for each drink containing alcohol

Take Alcohol Use Disorder Medications Regularly if Prescribed

- Typical medications:
  - Naltrexone
  - Acamprosate
  - Disulfiram
  - Gabapentin

Find Support

- Go to Alcoholics Anonymous (AA) meetings and get an AA sponsor
- Go to regular therapy sessions
- Find a recovery buddy, such as a friend who does not drink
- Identify the person or resource you will call in case of withdrawal symptoms or other emergency (eg, an AA sponsor, your doctor or on-call provider, 988)
  - In an emergency, I will call:

  _____

Identify Your Drinking Triggers and Alternative Activities

- My drinking triggers are:

  _____

  - Common triggers: HALT situations (Hungry, Angry, Lonely, Tired), boredom, sitting and watching TV

- My alternative activities are:

  _____

  - Common alternatives: Hobbies, exercise, renewed focus on work, volunteer activities, helping others in recovery (eg, in AA meetings)

www.ingramcontent.com/pod-product-compliance
Lightning Source LLC
Chambersburg PA
CBHW042342030426
42335CB00030B/3432